THE BASICS of

MISTAKE-PROOFING

MICHAEL R. BEAUREGARD
RAYMOND J. MIKULAK
ROBIN E. McDERMOTT

QUALITY RESOURCES.
A Division of The Kraus Organization Limited

Most Quality Resources books are available at quantity discounts when purchased in bulk. For more information contact:

Special Sales Department
Quality Resources
A Division of The Kraus Organization Limited
902 Broadway
New York, NY 10010
212-979-8600
800-247-8519

Printed in the United States of America

01 00 99 98 97   10 9 8 7 6 5 4 3 2 1

ISBN 0-527-76327-6

Contents

PREFACE

In 1983, I had the opportunity to live in Japan for six months and study the Toyota Production System under the tutelage of Taiichi Ohno, creator of the system. I expected to see lots of control charts for monitoring processes. In all of the companies in the Toyota system that I visited, I saw less than 10 control charts! What I saw instead was a tremendous emphasis on process engineering and process simplification. Although there were few control charts, among the many techniques I learned were kanbans, andons, SMED (single minute exchange of die), Taguchi methods, and this thing the Japanese engineers called poka-yoke. In my Japanese dictionary, poka-yoke translates to fool-proofing. My tutors, perhaps recognizing that their operators were not fools at all, translated it as mistake-proofing.

As I learned to apply the techniques to which I was being exposed, the one that we applied over and over was poka-yoke. After a while, it dawned on me that mistake-proofing wasn't new to me at all. I had learned to mistake-proof shortly after I graduated from college and started working for a large chemical manufacturer. The plant I worked in had a tremendous emphasis on safety. As a shift engineer, if a safety incident occurred, whether there was an injury or not, it was my responsibility to make sure a thorough investigation of the incident took place. From the investigation, we generated ideas and implemented process changes and procedures to make sure the incident couldn't happen again. We were mistake-proofing the process, using many of the same techniques described in this book, from a safety standpoint.

After this realization, it struck me that in all of my exposure to mistake-proofing from a safety standpoint, I had never thought of using the same approach and the same techniques to mistake-proof processes for the intermittent quality and productivity problems we had.

After I returned to the U.S., I found that most companies approached mistake-proofing the same way; as a safety tool. Mistake-proofing wasn't applied to improving manufacturing or service processes. In most companies, this focus on mistake-proofing as only a safety tool remained that way for years. Today, however, the use of mistake-proofing is changing. I'm glad to see mistake-proofing coming into the mainstream of process improvement. This is due mainly to the U.S. automotive industry's supplier improvement efforts and more recently by its inclusion into the QS-9000 Quality System Requirements.

This book aims to meet the needs of the enlightened engineers, managers, supervisors, and operators who recognize the need to mistake-proof their processes. It is also aimed to meet the needs of those who are strictly looking to meet the QS-9000 requirements. I can only speculate as to which group will be successful with mistake-proofing in the long run.

Michael R. Beauregard
January 1997

INTRODUCTION

Mistakes seem to happen at the worst time. At work, just before a critical shipment, an inadvertent mistake causes the entire shipment to be rejected. Or at home, just before leaving for a long-anticipated vacation, "Murphy's Law" intervenes, and a series of seemingly avoidable mistakes causes a delay.

Can we defeat Murphy's Law? Can we eliminate these costly mistakes? The answer is Yes! Mistakes can be eliminated by using mistake-proofing tools and techniques. Mistake-proofing will put an end to many of the repetitive, costly mistakes that rob us of time and money both at work and at home.

Making It Impossible to Make a Mistake

At its best, mistake-proofing is a technique for making it impossible to make mistakes. Mistake-proofing is accomplished by making permanent changes to equipment, operations, or procedures that eliminate opportunities for errors or provide an immediate signal if a mistake occurs.

Poka-Yoke Means Mistake-Proofing

The Japanese term for mistake-proofing is poka-yoke. Poka-yoke is pronounced *poe-ka-yo-kay*. A talented Japanese engineer, Shigeo Shingo coined the term and popularized the concepts in both Japan and the United States. As you learn about the basics of mistake-proofing, you will recognize mistake-proofing as the application of common sense, elegant in its

1

simplicity. Poka-yoke, or mistake-proofing, is the modern-day version of old-fashioned "Yankee ingenuity."

The Premise of Mistake-Proofing

Mistake-proofing is based on the premise that most defects are caused by human error. This is not to suggest that the errors are necessarily intentional, but rather that they are due to many different factors depending on the situation in which the error was made. Mistake-proofing techniques focus on taking the "human factor" out of making or doing something by replacing repetitive tasks or actions that require concentration and memory with tasks that are impossible to do any way but the right way. This does not mean that "thinking" is being taken out of the job, but rather that your time and mind are now free to pursue more creative and value-adding activities without the fear of making a mistake.

Zero Defects

Mistake-proofing works best when the quality objective is zero defects, because that forces us to think about improvement in a very different way. For example, reducing defects from 3 percent to 2 percent is relatively simple compared to eliminating defects altogether. Completely eliminating defects requires a different way of thinking about improving the process beyond working harder and being more conscious—it requires mistake-proofing.

Many think that zero defects is so implausible that it shouldn't be a goal. Yet isn't that what every organization's safety program strives to do—go to zero accidents? And isn't an accident just a serious defect? Just like we focus on mistake-proofing processes to eliminate the chance of an accident, we can focus on mistake-proofing to eliminate quality and productivity defects.

Examples of Mistake-Proofing in Everyday Life

The idea of mistake-proofing may seem foreign, but examples of mistake-proofing are all around us and we benefit from them everyday. Here are just a few examples:

- Auto shut-off irons so we cannot make the mistake of leaving the iron on all day.

- Automatic sinks in public facilities so the water cannot be left on when someone walks away.

- Coffee makers that stop brewing when the pot is removed.

- Circuit breakers that trip when they are overloaded.

- Electric heaters that turn off when they fall over.

- Car lights that shut off automatically.

- Audio/video tapes and computer disks that have an overwrite protector tab.

All of these product have been designed to make it impossible to make mistakes when using them. You can probably think of many more products that you use everyday that have mistake-proofing components built into them. How much do you depend on these mistake-proofing techniques? How much have you come to rely on mistake-proofing being built into the products you buy?

The Basics of Mistake-Proofing

Chapter 1
WHY MISTAKES ARE MADE

Most mistakes certainly are not intentional. Mistakes typically occur because of the complexity of a process. Even a seemingly simple manufacturing operation is complex in terms of the many variables that go into it.

Take, for example, the process of drilling a hole in a steel forging. The variables in that process include the grade of the steel, the drill speed, tool wear, the angle of the drill bit, where on the forging the hole is being drilled, the drilling technique the operator uses, and so on. After you consider all of these variables, it is no wonder that a hole drilled in each of the 10 different forgings may all turn out differently.

However, if you were a customer of this process, you would want, and would expect, every forging to be almost exactly the same. After all, if you are using the forging in your process to make, for example, a high-strength fitting, you need consistency in the forgings to assure consistency in your products.

Chances are that the processes you work in are at least as complicated as the process for drilling forgings. This means that there are probably lots of variables in your process, and therefore, many opportunities for mistakes.

Mistake-Proofing Eliminates Variables

Mistake-proofing reduces the variables, or choices, in a process, thereby reducing the opportunities for mistakes. For example, without mistake-proofing, you might have five options to choose among to get something done. One of those options is the right way and any other is the wrong way. With mistake-proofing techniques, there are no options from which the operator must choose. There is only one way, and that's the right way, to do something.

Chapter 2
ARE MISTAKES UNAVOIDABLE?

There are two schools of thought when it comes to mistakes. The first is that mistakes are inevitable and you need to learn how to live with them. This type of thinking is not productive in a mistake-proofing effort as it will almost always lead to failure.

The second school of thought is that mistakes can and must be eliminated. Although this thinking alone does not result in a mistake-proofing solution, it will enable more creative approaches to achieving zero defects.

The Mistake-Proofing Mind-Set

The right mind-set is an important component in the mistake-proofing process. Some of the traps people fall into that can derail mistake-proofing efforts include thinking the following:

- Inspection will always be necessary.

- People are "only human" and therefore will always make some level of mistakes.

- There is variation in everything, so there's no sense in trying to eliminate it.

- All operators have their own way of doing things and there's no way to change that.

Let's look at how each of these can hinder mistake-proofing efforts.

Inspection Is Necessary

If you're someone who feels inspection will always be necessary, ask yourself, "Why?" Chances are your answer is, "Because mistakes will always be made." What if that wasn't true? What if mistakes weren't always made? What if everything was always made right the first time? Then inspection wouldn't be necessary. That's the point we want to get to with mistake-proofing, because inspection is not the best way to assure quality—it adds costs and not value to the product. In addition, it is not 100 percent effective.

People Are "Only Human"

Often in manufacturing, you hear mistakes justified with the comment, "People are only human; mistakes are going to happen." That thinking justifies the purpose of mistake-proofing: to help reduce the human factors involved in correctly manufacturing a product by making it impossible to do something the wrong way.

There Is Variation in Everything

We've already mentioned the many variables that go into manufacturing a product. Mistake-proofing techniques are designed to reduce the opportunities for variation—especially special causes of variation that produce outliers—from creeping into a process by reducing or eliminating the number of variables in the process.

All Operators Have Their Own Way of Doing Things

There's a time for creativity in a job and there's a time for consistency. Most manufacturing operations require consistency and depend on operators following established procedures. Mistake-proofing techniques build adherence to the proper procedures right into the process. This will ensure consistency between operators.

Mistakes Can Be Eliminated

When engaging in a mistake-proofing effort, it is necessary to have the attitude that *mistakes can be eliminated*. This positive attitude will open the mind to considering previously unthought-of ways to eliminate mistakes. Once there is a recognition that mistakes can be eliminated, the opportunities for mistake-proofing will be endless. This will reduce dependence on inspection and will result in lower operating costs and higher quality.

Chapter 3
WHAT IS MISTAKE-PROOFING?

Mistake-proofing is actually a form of 100 percent inspection, although it is very different from traditional inspection.

Traditional inspection of a product is usually a separate step, completely unrelated to the manufacture of the product. With mistake-proofing, *the inspection process is part of the manufacturing process.* This is because the operator or user is usually the best inspector.

To illustrate the difference between traditional inspection and mistake-proofing, let's look at the example of a sheet-metal stamping operation. Five holes of varying sizes are punched into a 6¼" × 6½" piece of metal. Two problems continuously occur in this process. First, because there is only a ¼" difference between the long and short side of the part, it is often stamped in the wrong direction. Second, even if the part is put into the punch press in the right direction, there was no way to assure that it is lined up correctly so that the holes are punched in the right place on the part.

If the operation was using a traditional final inspection focus, either the operator or an inspector would check the finished part to determine if it was punched correctly. The problem with this approach is that the mistake has already been made. If the part is wrong, it will either have to be scrapped or reworked. The type of feedback in a traditional inspection process is shown in Figure 1.

Figure 1. Feedback process with traditional inspection.

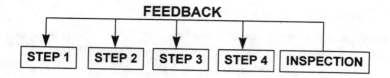

With mistake-proofing techniques, however, mistakes can be made impossible, eliminating the need for traditional inspection. There are probably several ways to mistake-proof this process. One of the easiest is to put a three-sided jig on the stamping machine into which the part will fit. If the part does not fit, the operator knows that it has been placed in the wrong direction. In addition, to ensure that the part is all the way in the jig, a sensor can be put on the back wall that will not allow the press to operate until contact is made with the part. In essence, the jig and sensor become the "inspector" built right into the process. The way feedback is provided in a mistake-proofed process is shown in Figure 2.

The Basics of Mistake-Proofing

Figure 2. Inspection feedback in a mistake-proofed process.

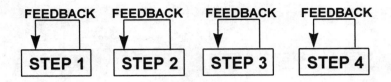

Production and inspection often become one and the same with the use of mistake-proofing techniques. That's what we mean when we say that mistake-proofing is a type of 100 percent inspection.

Chapter 4
HOW TO MISTAKE-PROOF

There are many avenues by which mistake-proofing can be achieved. To determine the right approach for your process, you must consider three concepts:

- The *purpose* for the mistake-proofing.

- The desired *outcome* of the mistake-proofing.

- The mistake-proofing *method* that is best for the situation.

Let's take a look at each of these in more detail. A summary of the concepts is found in Table 1 at the end of this chapter.

Purpose

There are two purposes for mistake-proofing:

- **Prevention**: To prevent a mistake from happening.

- **Detection**: To immediately identify when a mistake has occurred.

Prevention is obviously a more proactive approach to mistake-proofing compared to detection, which is more reactive and after-the-fact.

Outcome

One of four outcomes can result when a mistake is detected or is about to happen in a mistake-proofed process:

1. Control
2. Shutdown
3. Warning
4. Sensory alert.

Let's take a look at each of these in more detail.

Control

A control outcome self-corrects the process. This is the most desirable outcome with mistake-proofing because it provides immediate feedback and self-correction so that there is little or no disruption to the process.

A simple example of control involves electrical outlets. A 220-volt outlet is a different size and configuration than a 120-volt outlet. A 120-volt plug won't fit in. This controls the possibility of someone mistakenly plugging a 120-volt appliance into a 220-volt outlet.

Shutdown

A shutdown outcome triggers the process to shutdown when a mistake occurs. Although this type of outcome may result in loss of production, it also immediately stops any more mistakes from occurring.

A familiar example of shutdown is the automatic shut-off iron. This feature, now standard on many irons, prevents a potential fire by shutting off the iron after a set number of minutes without use.

Warning

A warning outcome signals the operator or user that a mistake or error has occurred or is about to occur.

The buzzer that sounds when a car is started and the driver hasn't fastened his or her seatbelt is an example of a warning outcome. The buzzer is an automatic signal to the driver, but by itself it does not assure safety. It is up to the individual receiving the warning to take action to avoid the mistake (in this case, a fatal or serious injury when the car is involved in an accident) from occurring or from getting worse. Distinctions between this type of outcome and control and shutdown will be discussed shortly.

Sensory Alert

A sensory alert is similar to a warning outcome in that it is up to the operator to take action when the signal is received. However, with the sensory alert, the operator is actually initiating the signal once the mistake is sensed through sight, sound, touch, smell, or taste. (This differs from warning outcomes, which produce a signal that has been automatically initiated by the process.)

An example of a sensory alert can be found in the small-parts machining industry. Many manufacturers use eggcrates for shipping small parts to prevent damage from scratches and nicks. Another benefit of the eggcrates is that they have a fixed number of holes in which parts can be placed. This makes it easy to ensure the right number of parts is shipped without a lot of nonvalue-adding counting of parts. For example, if an eggcrate has 30 holes and one is not filled, then the operator can quickly see (sense) the mistake in the number being shipped.

The difference between sensory alert and the other outcomes is that it requires operator diligence to sense the alert. In other words, the alert is not automatic. The operator must see that one part is missing and must take action to correct the mistake.

Which Is the Best Outcome?

To determine which is the best type of outcome when mistake-proofing, you need to consider how the outcome is triggered, what happens as a result of that trigger, and the potential cost and payback.

The outcome can be triggered either automatically or by the operator sensing the mistake. Control, shutdown, and warning are all the result of automatic triggers, whereas sensory alerts require that the operator sense the mistake. Obviously, the more effective trigger is the automatic trigger because it does not rely on operator diligence.

The Basics of Mistake-Proofing

Compulsory and Discretionary Action

Once the mistake is triggered, the action taken can be either compulsory or discretionary. A compulsory action gives the operator no choice in the outcome, whereas a discretionary action requires the operator to take action to fix the mistake or prevent other mistakes from occurring. Again, with mistake-proofing, we are trying to eliminate the reliance on operator diligence—compulsory results are more effective and, therefore, more desirable.

When determining the best mistake-proofing approach, it is helpful to think of the outcomes as being on a relative scale of effectiveness from 0 to 10 (see Figure 3). Although many factors must be taken into consideration when deciding on

Figure 3. Scale of mistake-proofing outcomes.

Relative Mistake-Proofing Power	Method	Trigger	Results
10 HIGH	Control	Automatic	Compulsory
9			
8			
7			
6	Shutdown		
5			
4			
3	Warning		Discretionary
2			
1	Sensory Alert	Operator Dependent	
0 LOW			

the best way to mistake-proof a process—e.g., cost, return on investment or payback, and effect on production—the scale helps focus the mistake-proofing team in the right direction.

Method

There is an unlimited number of tools and techniques that can be used for mistake-proofing. It helps to think of the various methods in terms of how they detect mistakes or potential mistakes. Shigeo Shingo, in his book *Study of "Toyota" Production System from Industrial Engineering Viewpoint*, identifies three broad categories of mistake-proofing methods: (1) contact, (2) performance step, and (3) fixed-value. We have added a fourth category that we call "making it easy to do it right."

Contact, performance step, and fixed-value mistake-proofing methods are process-initiated. Making it easy to do it right involves a series of operator-initiated, mistake-reduction techniques. Some people would not include mistake-reduction techniques in a discussion of mistake-proofing methods. However, our experience is that mistake-reduction methods can be effective when the cost or technical feasibility of true mistake-proofing methods is prohibitive.

Because there is overlap between the various methods, it is best to think of the method categories from a conceptual standpoint. In other words, use them to help you determine the method, but don't spend a lot of time trying to figure out into which category the method falls. What's important is that the process has been mistake-proofed, not that a specific method has been used.

Contact

Contact methods involve physical contact being made between two or more things. Electrical outlets use physical shape and contact with that shape to prevent the wrong-voltage appliances from being plugged in.

Another example, shown in Figure 4, is a guide pin on a mold for plastic parts. By having the contact of the guide pin protruding from one- half of the mold into a hole in the other half, the molder ensures the two mold halves are fitted properly when the mold is placed in a press. If the mold halves were not aligned properly, they could be damaged or destroyed the first time the press was run.

Figure 4. Mold with guide pin and hole.

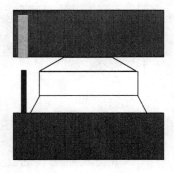

Performance Step

Performance step methods involve monitoring steps that are being performed and triggering an outcome if the step isn't performed correctly. For example, if a part must go through four different operations in a cell, a light and alarm buzzer may be set up to signal when one of the operations is skipped.

Another example of the use of the performance step method is in the final assembly of a CD-ROM in which seven screws of various sizes hold the equipment together. The seven screws can be stored in bins with photoelectric switches. When a screw is removed, the beam is broken. The part cannot move on to the next operation until the beam is broken on all seven bins. This is shown in Figure 5.

Figure 5. Screw bins with photoelectric switches.

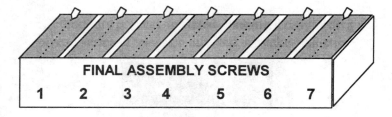

Fixed-value

Fixed-value methods involve setting specific values that trigger a mistake-proofing outcome and having the process count up to that trigger. For example, if an operator has to package

12 three-ring binders in a box, a photoelectric eye and programmable controller could be used to count how many binders the operator has picked up. Until 12 have been picked up and moved through the photoelectric beam, the box is blocked from going down the conveyor.

Another example of the use of fixed-value is a weigh counter, which is a special type of scale that will tell you how many parts are on the scale based on the weight of one part. Nameplate manufacturers use weigh scales, like the one in Figure 6, to make sure the right number of nameplates is packaged in every bag. For example, if their customer wants 100 nameplates per bag, they will set the scale so that a warning goes off if too few or too many nameplates are in the bag.

Figure 6. Fixed-value weigh scale.

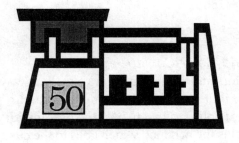

Making It Easy To Do It Right

There may be times that true, process-initiated mistake-proofing is not possible. Sometimes it may be too costly, and other times control, shutdown, or warning devices just might not be appropriate for a specific process. In these cases, mistake-proofing aids can make it easy to do it right.

Some of the more common ways to make it easy to do something right include:

- Colors and color-coding.

- Shapes.

- Symbols.

- Operator initiated auto-detection.

- Other tools.

We'll look at each of these more detail.

Colors and Color-Coding

Use of colors and color-coding are excellent ways to make it easy to do things right. For example, multipart forms often make use of color-coding to help the user identify which part of the form is the original, which goes to the customer, which goes to accounting, and so on.

Another example of color-coding is used by some computer manufacturers to make it easy for their customers to hook up their computers. They assign different colors to the various ports and plugs on the back of the computer, which then can be easily matched up with the correct cable because it, too, has been color-coded.

Even some zipper-type plastic bags are color-coded, with one side of the seal being blue and the other yellow. The user knows that the bag is sealed because the two strips interlock and turn green.

None of these color-coding examples are 100 percent mistake-proofing, however, because they are not making it impossible to do something the wrong way. Instead, the use of colors and color-coding just make it easier to do things right in cases where it is not practical, feasible, or cost effective to 100 percent mistake-proof the process.

Symbols

Like colors and shapes, symbols can make it easier to do something right. Symbols can be used as icons or visual identifiers that enable the user to make quick matches with a high rate of accuracy, although they still do not offer a mistake-free solution.

Shapes

Different shapes associated with different conditions can also help make it easy to do things right. There are a variety of ways that shapes can be used when mistake-proofing is not possible.

One example of using shapes can be found in offices that deal with a lot of different forms. If there is a problem with the various forms getting mixed up, each type of form can be notched in a unique spot on the form. When the forms are in a stack, it will be easy to tell which don't belong because they will not be notched in the right place.

Shapes also can be used to keep track of hand tools in a workshop or maintenance department. By painting a pegboard with silhouettes of each of the tools and then hanging the tools over the silhouettes, it will be easy to determine if any tools are missing.

Operator-Initiated Autodetection

Operator-initiated autodetection devices automatically find mistakes for the operator or user. These devices, however, must be activated by the operator or they will not function. This is what distinguishes these techniques from true mistake-proofing.

For example, word processing programs have spell-check features that help the user identify misspelled words so they can be corrected. However, in many programs, it is up to the operator to initiate the spell-checking feature, and because of this, the spell checking feature is not considered mistake-proofing. Newer word processing packages do build mistake-proofing components into the spell-checking feature. For example, they have a database of commonly misspelled words along with the correct spelling. Anytime the commonly misspelled word is recognized as being misspelled, it is automatically corrected without the user even knowing it. Another mistake-proofing technique built into spell-checkers today is that misspelled words are automatically underlined. The purpose of this mistake-proofing feature, however, is detection, not prevention.

Other Tools That Make It Easy to Do It Right

Other tools that help make it easy to do something right include:

- **Checklists.** Checklists serve as useful reminders, providing that they are precisely followed. One of the problems with checklists, however, is that when they are used in processes that are performed regularly, they become annoying paperwork that is often filled out after the fact from memory rather than throughout the process as a memory aid. For this reason, it is best to use checklists on processes that are performed infrequently.

- **Forms.** Forms, like checklists, lose their effectiveness the more frequently they are used. Once people become familiar with the form, they may slip into the habit of just filling in the blanks rather than using it to guide them through their process.

- **Procedures.** If used, procedures can help bring consistency and uniformity to a process. However, a bad procedure may result in bad products. In addition, there is nothing to prevent someone from deviating from a procedure.

- **Simplified Workflows.** Complicated workflows invite mistakes because they are difficult to follow, involve numerous hand-offs, and contain many opportunities for mistakes. A simplified workflow is easier to follow, reduces the number of hand-offs, and greatly reduces the opportunities for mistakes.

Table 1. Recap of Mistake-Proofing Concepts.

Purpose	Outcomes	Methods
Prevention	Control	Contact
Detection	Shutdown	Performance step
	Warning	Fixed-value
	Sensory alert	Making it easy to do it right

Chapter 5
WHEN WON'T
MISTAKE-PROOFING WORK?

Although mistake-proofing systems are designed to prevent mistakes, sometimes a mistake happens even with the system in place because of some type of malfunction or breakdown in the system. The two common reasons that mistake-proofing systems break down are (1) the system is intentionally disabled or (2) there is a mechanical, electrical, or other type of nonhuman malfunction in the system.

Disabling Mistake-Proofing Systems

Although mistake-proofing systems are designed to make it impossible to make mistakes, often the implementation of the system relies on operators putting them in place during setup. For example, most machines have guards to protect operators from injuries. A guard on a printing press, for example, may make it impossible to put a finger or hand in a pinch point. However, that mistake-proofing technique requires that the operator puts the guard in place.

This brings up an important point about mistake-proofing—mistake-proofing techniques must be used to be effective. Although this is an obvious statement, it is necessary to emphasize because it is not unusual to see mistake-proofing systems overridden or disabled.

Two primary reasons that mistake-proofing systems are overridden are willful volition and malicious intent.

Willful Volition

Sometimes operators will deliberately override a mistake-proofing system with only the best intentions in mind. When you ask these operators why they disabled the system, they may tell you that it slowed down production, created other problems or mistakes, or restricted their access to areas in the equipment they need to get to quickly. Very often when you hear these types of comments, it is because the operator was not involved in the mistake-proofing process and has become a sort of victim of mistake-proofing rather than a beneficiary.

No one knows the job better than the person who works on it everyday. To mistake-proof a process without his or her input is only asking for problems. Even the best mistake-proofing solutions will be difficult to implement if they are being forced on people who have no say in how they should be set up. Involving the process operators in the mistake-proofing effort will enable them to take ownership for the solutions, and they will help implement those solutions rather than work against them.

Malicious Intent

Although it infrequently happens, sometimes mistake-proofing systems are overridden or disabled intentionally to sabotage the process. Mistake-proofing techniques will not stop that rare malicious employee that is out to harm the process or product. In these cases, disciplinary action must be taken to resolve the problem.

The possibility of malicious intent supports the need for procedures that are well-documented and well-understood. With these, operators should have a clear understanding of how the mistake-proofing system should be used as well as the consequences of not properly using them. Then, if a mistake-proofing system is overridden, quick and consistent disciplinary action must be taken to maintain the integrity of the system.

Malfunctioning Mistake-Proofing Systems

Many of the examples we have reviewed have been mechanical approaches to mistake-proofing, such as the electrical plug with one prong larger than the other to make it impossible to insert the plug incorrectly. These types of mistake-proofing systems are reasonably reliable because of their simplicity.

However, in recent years, many mistake-proofing systems have included electronic sensing devices and other equipment that, because of their complex nature, can malfunction for a many reasons, including lack of proper care, technical failures, and electrical surges and spikes.

Preventing Malfunctions

Ideally, mistake-proofing systems themselves should be mistake-proofed. However, this may not always be practical, feasible, or cost-effective. Therefore, it is important to include regular checks, at least daily or at the start of each shift, to ensure that the mistake-proofing system is working properly.

Chapter 6
PRACTICAL, FEASIBLE, AND COST-EFFECTIVE MISTAKE-PROOFING

One mistake-proofing solution can save a company hundreds, thousands, or even tens of thousands of dollars. On the other hand, there will be some cost associated with implementing a mistake-proofing solution as well. Many mistake-proofing techniques are inexpensive and easy to implement, but others can be costly, disruptive to production, and may have a payback period that is unacceptable to the organization. Therefore, when developing mistake-proofing solutions, it is important to make sure the solution is practical, feasible, and cost-effective.

Practical Mistake-Proofing Solutions

Practical mistake-proofing solutions are those that seem to make sense given the situation. For example, if you are planning to install a vision system that you must totally customize to try to get it to work in the application, it may not be practical unless you're an optics engineer. Other examples of impractical solutions: If your facility does not have electronic systems in place, it would not be practical to use a mistake-proofing system based on electronics. If no one in your facility is computer-literate, a mistake-proofing approach based on the use on computers would not be practical, even though it may be both feasible and cost-effective.

Feasible Mistake-Proofing Solutions

A mistake-proofing solution also must be technically feasible. For this reason, it might help to get engineering input when the solutions are being developed. In addition, proving the mistake-proofing solution on paper or in a simulated model could identify some less obvious problems with the design before time and money are invested in a solution that is not operational.

Cost-Effective Mistake-Proofing Solutions

A cost-effective mistake-proofing solution is one that you can afford. The difficulty here is capturing exactly what the savings will be because many of the costs of not mistake-proofing a process are intangible. For example, if a process is not mistake-proofed, it could result in defective product, which results in an obvious cost to the company. However, if the defective product reaches the customer, there are other costs as well that are less easy to measure, such as the cost of a dissatisfied customer or the cost of a potential injury as a result of the defective product.

There is a great deal of information available today on how to conduct a cost-benefit analysis, so we won't go into that in depth in this book. Instead, we will look at it conceptually.

Payback

Most companies currently require a financial payback within a specified time frame for all capital expenditures. Many mistake-proofing solutions don't require capital expenditures, so payback won't be an issue. However, if the solution does involve a capital expenditure, a payback analysis will help ensure that the benefit outweighs the cost.

To determine payback, you must establish the cost of the mistakes to the organization on a monthly basis. The cost for the mistake-proofing solution then would be compared to the cost of the mistakes to determine how long it will take to recoup the cost of implementing the solution.

For example, if a certain type of mistake is costing $500 a month and the mistake-proofing solution costs $1,500, the single payback period is three months. Many companies today require a six-month to one-year single payback. Because this solution fits in those guidelines, it would be implemented. On the other hand, if a mistake is costing $100 a month and the mistake-proofing solution costs $1,500, the single payback period is 15 months. This may be longer than a company is willing to wait for a payback and therefore the solution would not be implemented. Tables 2 and 3 show scenarios of the short- and long-payback periods, respectively.

Table 2. Scenario A: Short Payback Period (Implement the mistake-proofing solution).

Monthly Cost of Mistake	$500
Cost for Mistake-Proofing	$1,500
Payback Period	$1,500 ÷ $500 = 3 months

Table 3. Scenario B: Long Payback Period (DO NOT implement the mistake-proofing solution).

Monthly Cost of Mistake	$100
Cost for Mistake-Proofing	$1,500
Payback Period	$1,500 ÷ $100 = 15 months

As has already been noted, many mistake-proofing solutions are relatively inexpensive (under $1,000) and, in many cases, payback will not be an issue. If payback does become an issue, then other mistake-proofing solutions should be employed.

Chapter 7
MISTAKE-PROOFING STEPS

Mistake-proofing doesn't just happen. Like any other quality improvement effort, it takes teamwork and problem-solving skills. It is best to use a planned and methodical approach to mistake-proofing. Key steps in the mistake-proofing process include:

Step 1: Identify problems

Step 2: Prioritize problems

Step 3: Find the root cause

Step 4: Create solutions

Step 5: Measure the results

We'll look at each of these steps in more detail in the following sections.

Step 1: Identify Problems

The first step in a mistake-proofing effort is to identify problems. In this stage, you shouldn't be concerned whether you have an effective mistake-proofing technique to solve the problem. Those ideas will come later. There are several ways to identify mistake-proofing opportunities. They include:

- Brainstorming

- Customer returns

- Defective-parts analysis

- Scrap analysis

- Process error reports

- Failure mode and effects analysis (FMEA)

- Reliable data.

Brainstorming

Brainstorming is a technique used to generate a large number of ideas in a short period of time with input from many people. It provides an excellent way to develop a list of potential mistake-proofing projects.

There are many different ways to brainstorm depending on the objective of the brainstorming session. A round-robin approach works best with mistake-proofing because it allows each person the opportunity to express their ideas, while keeping the energy level high.

The Basics of Mistake-Proofing

It helps to review the rules of round-robin-style brainstorming with the group before the brainstorming session begins. They include the following:

- Do not comment on, judge, or critique ideas as they are offered.

- Encourage creative and offbeat ideas.

- A large amount of ideas is the goal.

- Evaluate ideas later.

Customer Returns

Customer returns provide an excellent outside source of ideas for mistake-proofing opportunities. What makes customer returns a unique source of ideas is that not only do they point to process mistake-proofing opportunities, but they provide ideas for mistake-proofing how the product is used by the customer. Use the returns to help get customers involved in mistake-proofing solutions.

Process Error Reports

A process error is a mistake made by the process. The process can be a human process or it can be an automated process. Gathering data on types and frequency of process errors will provide sound evidence of where mistake-proofing techniques are most needed.

Defective-Parts Analysis

A defective-parts analysis identifies the type and frequency of product defects. Like the process error report, a defective-parts analysis can identify where mistake-proofing applications are most needed in the manufacturing process. It is helpful to use a prioritizing technique, such as the Pareto diagram shown in Figure 7, when conducting a defective parts analysis.

Scrap Analysis

While a scrap analysis may seem similar to a defective-parts analysis, scrap analysis looks at wasted materials throughout the process, not just at the end of the process—after the part is made—as is done with defective-parts analysis.

Figure 7. Pareto diagram of a defective parts analysis.

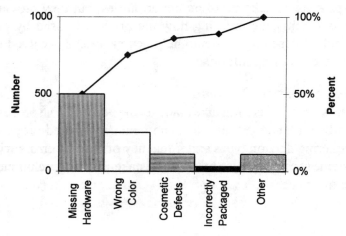

The Basics of Mistake-Proofing

Failure Mode and Effects Analysis (FMEA)

A failure mode and effects analysis (FMEA) is a systematic review of potential product and process problems, usually prior to the startup of a new process. With an FMEA, a team of people knowledgeable about a process predict:

- What can go wrong with the process or product.

- What will be the effect.

- What the frequency and severity of the failure will be and what is the probability of detection.

Weights and points assigned to the frequency, severity, and probability then can be used to prioritize which failures will be targeted for mistake-proofing. FMEA is covered in more detail in the next chapter.

Reliable Data

It's important that the data used in this first step of the process be reliable data. If it is not, you be may using your limited resources to mistake-proof a process that doesn't need it nearly as much as a process that does but is being ignored.

Step 2: Prioritize Problems

There will no doubt be a long list of mistake-proofing opportunities identified in Step 1 of the mistake-proofing process. It is likely that there won't be enough people or resources to address all of the mistake-proofing opportunities at once. This means that the problems must be prioritized in some kind of order to ensure that the most critical problems are addressed first. The question is, "How do you determine the 'most critical problems'?"

There are several ways to go about prioritizing problems for mistake-proofing. They include:

- **Frequency of Occurrence.** How often the problem is occurring. Obviously, if a problem rarely occurs, it probably won't be at the top of your mistake-proofing list unless the problem is very costly or if it could result in an injury to the operator or user.

- **Wasted Materials.** Another way to decide which opportunities to mistake-proof first is to consider the amount of wasted material or scrap associated with the problem. Because wasted material translates into wasted money, you will want to focus on the biggest material wastes first.

- **Rework Time.** Rework time is another consideration in prioritizing mistake-proofing opportunities. Like wasted materials, rework time means wasted money, so you should focus on those rework areas that are the most costly.

- **Detection Time/Cost.** Detection time is the time it takes to find mistakes. Sometimes defects are easy to find and take little time to surface. Other mistakes take more time to surface. Detection cost is the cost spent finding mistakes; in other words, the cost for inspection. Detection cost is distinguished from detection time because there may be a case where a mistake takes little time to find, but the inspection method is costly, for example, with destructive testing.

- **Overall Cost.** The overall cost of a mistake takes into account the costs already mentioned as well as other less tangible, but equally important costs, such as the cost of a lost customer or a product liability or warrantee issue.

Use the Pareto Principle

The Pareto Principle is a tool that can be used to prioritize problems. It is often referred to as the 80/20 rule, meaning that typically 80 percent of the problems can be solved with 20 percent of the effort. Using the Pareto Principle helps you focus on the vital few problems that are most costly to the organization, assuring you get the most bang for your mistake-proofing "buck."

To conduct a Pareto analysis of problems, you need to determine what criteria you will be using to evaluate problems. For example, are you going to look at problems in terms of their overall cost to the organization, the amount of rework they generate, or the cost of detecting the mistake? Let's say you decide to use rework as the criterion. You would assign

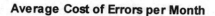

Figure 8. Pareto analysis of the cost of mistakes.

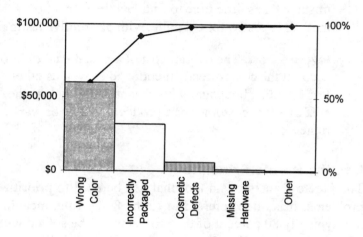

each type of mistake a category and then determine how much rework each category causes. The categories would be put in order from the highest level of rework to the least amount. If your objective is to reduce rework through mistake-proofing, it will now be obvious which of the mistake categories you should focus on first.

Figure 8 shows a Pareto diagram of the cost of mistakes on a monthly basis. The Pareto diagram makes it clear that the wrong color problem should be addressed first.

Step 3: Find the Root Cause

Don't use mistake-proofing to cover up problems or to treat symptoms. Use mistake-proofing to correct errors at their source. That is what is meant by, "find the root cause." When mistake-proofing is put in place to cover up problems that should be fixed, it creates, nonvalue-adding costs to the organization.

The Five W's and One H
It helps to consider the who, what, where, when, why, and how of a mistake when you are trying to get to its root cause. Here are some questions you should be asking yourself:

- **Who?** Who is experiencing the problem? Is it all people who work in the process or just some of them?

- **What?** What is the specific problem? What is its impact?

- **Where?** Where is the problem occurring? Where is the source or root cause of the problem? Where isn't the problem occurring?

- **When?** When does the problem occur? During certain times? Is there a cycle to the problem? When doesn't it occur?

- **Why?** Why do you think the problem occurs? Why doesn't it occur all the time? (Ask why five times to get to the root cause.)

- **How?** How many times has the problem occurred? How can the problem be mistake-proofed?

Step 4: Create Solutions

Make It Impossible to Do It Wrong
Use the techniques described—such as contact, performance step, and fixed-value—to develop mistake-proofing solutions that make it impossible to do something wrong. This step in the process requires creativity to think beyond the obvious. After all, if mistake-proofing solutions were obvious, everything would already be mistake-proofed!

Cost-Benefit Analysis
The cost-benefit analysis is used to determine exactly how long it will take to recover the cost of the solution. Refer to Chapter 7 to review how to conduct a cost-benefit analysis.

Step 5: Measure the Results

As with any improvement process, it is important to measure the results of the effort to determine if additional action is necessary.

Have Errors Been Eliminated?

To determine if errors have been eliminated, compare the current errors to the past errors before mistake-proofing. If it appears that the error is still there, you must find out why. If new errors have now arisen, they, too, should be tracked as they are candidates for future mistake-proofing.

What Is the Financial Impact?

Now is the time to go back and compare your cost-benefit analysis to the actual performance of the mistake-proofing solution. Has the expected benefit been achieved? This type of information is valuable not only to justify the current mistake-proofing efforts, but to justify mistake-proofing needs for the future. In addition, management will be looking for those bottom-line tangible results before they are willing to invest more money training and teaching others how to mistake-proof.

Typically, we have found mistake-proofing efforts yield a payback measured in weeks or possibly months, not years. The graph in Figure 9 shows the way one company tracked its savings after mistake-proofing efforts.

Figure 9. Tracking savings from mistake-proofing.

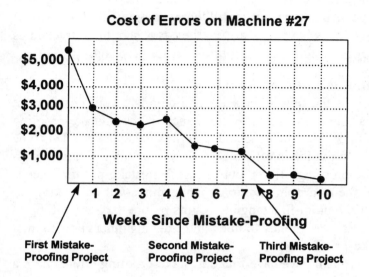

The Basics of Mistake-Proofing

Chapter 8
FMEA AND MISTAKE-PROOFING

Failure mode and effect analysis (FMEA) and mistake-proofing go hand in hand. An FMEA helps identify potential product and process problems in the design stage with the objective being to change product and/or process designs to eliminate the potential problems. Very often, the solution to a problem identified through an FMEA is a mistake-proofing solution. For more specific information on how to conduct an FMEA, we suggest you refer to *The Basics of FMEA* a companion book to *The Basics of Mistake-Proofing*. However, to help you understand the power of FMEA and how it can be used with mistake-proofing, we'll provide a brief overview of the process here.

Conducting an FMEA

The purposes of an FMEA for either a process or a product are to:

- Determine what can go wrong with the process or product.

- Anticipate what the effect(s) will be.

- Estimate the frequency, severity, and probability of the effect(s).

This is done through an in-depth analysis of the process or product. FMEAs are typically conducted by cross-functional teams of employees, some who have experience with the subject—for example, they have worked with similar products or processes and are familiar with the types of potential failures, scrap rates, and assembly problems that may occur—and others who have no experience with it. In this way, a variety of perspectives will be included in the FMEA project.

An FMEA begins with a brainstorming session where a list of all potential failures is developed. Next, the team determines the possible effects of those failures. This information is then used to evaluate the risk of failure. There are three criteria that are considered here:

1. *Severity*—the consequence of the failure should it occur.

2. *Occurrence*—the probability or frequency of the failure occurring.

3. *Detection*—the probability of the failure being detected before the impact of the effect is realized.

Each of these is rated on a scale of 1 to 10, with 1 being the lowest possible rating and 10 being the highest. Once the rating process is complete, a risk-priority number is assigned. The risk-priority number for each potential failure is simply the severity times the occurrence times the detection rating.

Failures with the highest risk-priority number are those on which the FMEA team concentrates. Although there are a variety of ways to reduce the risk-priority numbers, one of the most effective techniques is mistake-proofing. Table 4 shows an example of an FMEA worksheet.

Table 4. Example of an FMEA Worksheet.

Potential Problem	Effect(s)	Frequency	Severity	Detection	Total Score
Air hose clogs					
Gasket leaks					
Filter Fails					
Power cuts off					

Once improvements have been made to the process or product, a new rating is done for each of the improved items on the FMEA. The new ratings should be significantly lower than the old ratings, indicating that substantial improvements have been made.

Chapter 9
EXAMPLES OF LINKING
METHODS AND OUTCOMES

In most complex processes, multiple mistake-proofing methods and related outcomes are needed to ensure the process performs as desired. The following examples show how multiple combinations of methods/outcomes can be applied to the same process.

Example 1: Packaging Line for Greeting Cards

Situation
A high-volume manufacturer of greeting cards has elected to install an automated boxing and packaging line. Each box contains 20 cards and 20 envelopes. Two self-counting feeders load 10 envelopes, each followed by two more self-counting feeders loading 10 cards each into the box. The box is conveyed to a shrink-wrapping line before being conveyed to the shipping carton. See Figure 10 for a schematic of the line.

Criteria
- The line must fill and shrink-wrap one filled box every 20 seconds.

Figure 10. Schematic of packaging line.

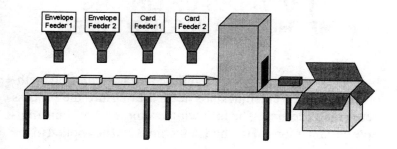

- All filled card boxes must have the correct count of cards and envelopes to be accepted.

- Boxes with incorrect counts must be isolated and diverted before the shrink-wrapping unit.

- The packaging line is to shut itself down if it repeatedly miscounts cards or envelopes.

- The packaging line is to shut itself down if it jams.

Mistake-Proofing Purpose

Prevention

- To ensure product with defective counts of cards or envelopes do not leave the process.

- To prevent the process from operating if major process deficiencies (e.g., no boxes, recurring feeder defects) occur.

Detection

- To identify any product-count error and isolate it from good product.

- To warn the process operator of intermittent and/or recurring process errors.

Mistake-Proofing Method/Outcome Combinations

The solutions used for this process involved three mistake-proofing methods (contact, performance step, and fixed-value) and three mistaking-proofing outcomes (shutdown, control, and warning).

- **Contact/Shutdown.** The process starts with an empty box. A direct-contact pressure switch is used to ensure the box has been delivered. If the box has not been delivered, the process shuts down.

- **Performance Step/Control.** If a feeder misfires (counts too few or two many cards or envelopes), the box is ejected from the line before the shrink-wrap unit.

- **Performance Step/Warning.** If a feeder misfires (counts too few or too many cards or envelopes), a warning light comes on to indicate that a box has been rejected. The light stays on until it is reset manually.

- **Fixed-Value/Shutdown.** If the same feeder misfires (counts too few or too many cards or envelopes) three times in a row, the line shuts down.

Example 2: Electronic-Circuit-Board Assembly

Situation

A captive electronic-circuit-board assembly operation is experiencing a rise in the level of errors in component placement and orientation. The process problem has lead to high rework costs, temporary initiation of 100 percent inspection, and difficulty in keeping up with production demands.

Criteria

- Correct circuit-board assembly, right the first time.

- Faster cycle times.

Mistake-Proofing Purpose

Prevention

- To use processing aids (kitting, locator) to assemble the circuit boards correctly the first time.

Detection

- To aid in locating an assembly error (overlays) before it leaves production.

Mistake-Proofing Method/Outcome Combinations

The solutions used for this process involve three mistake-proofing methods (performance step, fixed-value, and making it easy to do it right) and two mistake-proofing outcomes (control and sensory alert).

- **Fixed-Value/Control.** A "kitting" approach to component preparation was put in practice. Preselected kits of components were prepared. The correct number of components for the lot size to be produced was selected from stock and segregated by component type into bags. The bags were numbered in sequential assembly order. The assembly operator now had an accurate count of components. As the fixed-value of components was a match to the lot size, all components should be used with no shortages and none leftover.

- **Performance Step/Control.** A locator light device was employed to help place components correctly in the next sequential performance step. The locator unit is programmed to shine a light beam at the location of the next component to be place.

- **Making It Easy to Do It Right.** Transparent color overlays of the circuit board were made to compare the assembled board to the visual model. The overlay helps ensure the correct orientation and placement of parts and provides a sensory alert of potential defects to the operator.

Example 3: Loading Tanker with Liquid Paint

Situation

A producer of paint ships in bulk-tanker quantities to regional distribution and packaging facilities. The same equipment is used to manufacture several different colors of paint.

One of the most serious process issues is cross-color contamination of paint. The manufacturing process has tank cleaning and pipe flushing systems in place. See Figure 11.

Figure 11. Paint manufacturing cleaning system.

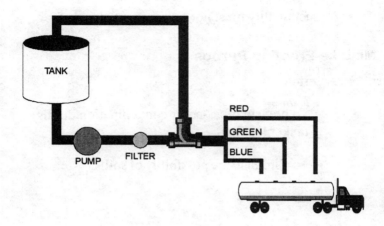

However, transferring the paint into tankers without contamination or spills occurring continues to be a source of concern. Tankers are loaded using a hose hooked up to the paint-holding-tank discharge pump. A different hose for each color of paint manufactured is used to minimize the potential of cross-color contamination.

Criteria

- There must be no cross-contamination of colors of paint.

- There must be no spills of paint.

- The tanker should be loaded within 2 hours.

- Product quality must not be not jeopardized.

Mistake-Proofing Purpose

Prevention

- To prevent cross-color contamination during tanker loading.

- To eliminate the possibility of spills.

Detection

- To warn the process operator (and shut down the process) if an unusual process operation occurs.

Mistake-Proofing Method/Outcome Combinations

The solutions used for this process involved two mistake-proofing methods (performance step and fixed-value) and three mistake-proofing outcomes (shutdown, control, and warning).

- **Performance Step/Control.** Eliminate the hoses. They don't mistake-proof the operation, are difficult to clean, and lead the spills whenever used. Modify the piping system. Include the tanker loading system in the cleaning system. Flush the tanker's transfer piping

The Basics of Mistake-Proofing

system back into the holding tank until the flushing fluid is clear.

- **Fixed-Value/Shutdown.** While the paint is metered into the tanker, overflows have occurred. Place a fluid- level control in the tanker during loading to ensure the tanker is not overfilled. If a predetermined fixed (high) level is reached, the level control would shut down the transfer pump.

- **Performance Step/Warning or Shutdown.** Add a pressure switch before the transfer pump. If the pressure is too high, it could indicate a plugged discharge filter. If the pressure dropped suddenly, it could indicate a break in the filter.

APPENDIX

List of Mistake-Proofing Process Tools[*]

Contact Detection Methods

Limit switches	Differential transformers	Trimetrons
Microswitches	Liquid level relays	Touch switches

Noncontact Methods

Dimension sensors	Positioning sensors
Fluid elements	Displacement sensors
Metal passage sensors	Tap sensors
Beam sensors	Color-marking sensors
Fiber sensors	Vibration sensors
Area sensors	Double-feed sensors
Photoelectric switches	Welding position sensors
Proximity detection measures	

Other Methods

(Detecting pressure, temperature, electric current, vibration, number of cycles, timing, and information transmission)

Pressure gages	Current Eyes	Meter relays
Vibration sensors	Counters	Fiber sensors
Thermometers	PLCs	Thermostats
Thermistors	Pressure-sensitive switches	

[*] Source: S. Shingo (1986). *Zero Quality Control: Source Inspection and the Poka-Yoke System*. Portland, OR: Productivity Press.

Related Resources

Kozak, R. J. and G. Krafcisin (1997). *Safety Management and ISO 9000/QS-9000: A Guide to Alignment and Integration.* New York: Quality Resources.

McDermott, R. E., R. J. Mikulak, and M. R. Beauregard (1996). *The Basics of* FMEA. New York: Quality Resources.

Osada, T. (1991). *The 5 S's: Five Keys to a Total Quality Environment.* Tokyo: Asian Productivity Association (distributed in the United States by Quality Resources, New York, NY).

Shingo, S. (1981). *Study of "Toyota" Production System From Industrial Engineering Viewpoint.* Tokyo: Japan Management Association.

Shingo, S. (1986). *Zero Quality Control: Source Inspection and the Poka-Yoke System.* Portland, OR: Productivity Press.

Awards

Shingo Prize for Excellence in Manufacturing. College of Business, Utah State University, Logan, UT 84322-3521. Tel: 801-750-2279. Fax: 801-750-3440. (This is an excellent source for examples of mistake-proofing and other quality improvement techniques.)